How to Be a Master of Yourself: A Guide to Master Your Skills and Be One

Josh Jones

Copyright Notice

Copyright © 2024 by Josh Jones. All rights reserved. No part of this publication may be reproduced, distributed, or transmitted in any form or by any means, including photocopying, recording, or other electronic or mechanical methods, without the prior written permission of the publisher, except in the case of brief quotations embodied in critical reviews and certain other noncommercial uses permitted by copyright law. For permission requests, write to the publisher, addressed "Attention: Permissions Coordinator," at the address provided.

Disclaimer

This book is intended for informational and educational purposes only. The views and opinions expressed herein are those of the author and do not necessarily reflect the official policy or position of any agency of the author's. All content provided is the author's opinion and is not intended as specific advice. Readers should consult appropriate professionals before making any significant decisions based on the content of this book.

To all who have ever felt lost on their path, may this book serve as a compass, guiding you towards the mastery of your own destiny.

In the quest to master self, a journey deep and true,
Through pages, words, and wisdom, a light begins to brew.
With every step and stumble, in shadows and in light,
This guide, a beacon, calling, through day and into night.
A mastery of mind and soul, where dreams are forged in fire,
Beyond the realms of doubt and fear, to higher ground aspire.
Each chapter a stepping stone, in rivers wide and deep,
Where knowledge flows like water, and wisdom's seeds we reap.
So take this book, this map of sorts, into your hands, your heart,
And find within its pages, the place where journeys start.
For mastery's not just a goal, but a path that's ever new,
"In mastering of self," it says, "you'll find the world anew."

Foreword

In the vast ocean of self-help and personal development literature, it's rare to come across a beacon of genuine insight and practical wisdom. "How to Be a Master of Yourself: A Guide to Master Your Skills and Be One," by Josh Jones, is one such beacon. It's an honor and a privilege to write this foreword for a book that I believe will illuminate the path for countless individuals seeking to navigate the complex journey of self-mastery.

Josh Jones has crafted a guide that transcends the ordinary by diving deep into the essence of what it means to truly master oneself. This book is not just a collection of advice; it is a meticulously designed journey that challenges, teaches, and inspires its readers to reach new heights of personal achievement and fulfillment.

From the moment I turned the first page, I was captivated by the depth of understanding and the clarity of vision that Josh brings to the table. His approach to mastering skills and integrating them into a cohesive sense of self is both innovative and deeply respectful of the individual's unique journey. Josh doesn't just tell you what to do; he walks with you, guiding you through the complexities of personal growth with empathy, expertise, and a clear-eyed focus on the end goal.

What sets this book apart is its holistic approach to mastery. Josh understands that to master oneself, one must look beyond the surface skills and delve into the deeper realms of mindset, emotional intelligence, and the often overlooked art of living a balanced and harmonious life. His chapters on mindfulness, overcoming obstacles, and integrating your skills offer invaluable insights into the process of becoming not just proficient in various areas of life, but truly unified and whole.

In a world where quick fixes and superficial solutions are all too common, "How to Be a Master of Yourself" stands out as a testament to the power of dedicated, thoughtful, and sustained effort. Josh Jones has not only provided a roadmap to mastery; he has also lit the torch that will guide us along the way.

As you embark on this journey with Josh as your guide, I encourage you to approach this book with an open heart and a willing spirit. The path to self-mastery is not always easy, but it is always worth it. And with "How to Be a Master of Yourself" in your hands, you have everything you need to start your journey on the right foot.

To your journey,
Jarod Hogs

Embarking on a journey of self-mastery is akin to setting sail into the vast, uncharted waters of the self. It requires courage, resilience, and an unwavering commitment to delve into the depths of one's own being, exploring the myriad facets that compose the human experience. This journey is not for the faint-hearted, nor is it a path that promises quick fixes or shortcuts. Instead, it offers something far more valuable: a profound understanding of oneself and the acquisition of skills that empower an individual to lead a life of purpose, fulfillment, and harmony.

The essence of mastering oneself lies not in the accumulation of external accolades or achievements, but in the quiet, persistent work of inner development. It is a process that demands introspection, the willingness to confront one's own limitations, and the courage to step beyond them. This book is born out of the belief that every individual holds within them the potential for greatness, not as defined by society, but as sculpted by the deepest truths of their own soul.

Mastery of oneself is a multifaceted endeavour. It encompasses the mastery of one's thoughts, emotions, actions, and reactions. It involves cultivating a mindset that embraces growth, fostering emotional intelligence that enriches one's interactions with others, and developing a suite of skills that enable one to navigate the complexities of life with grace and competence. However, the journey does not stop at the self. True mastery extends its reach into the world, manifesting through meaningful contributions, the creation of lasting relationships, and the ability to inspire and uplift those around us.

At its core, the pursuit of self-mastery is a deeply personal quest, yet it is also universally relevant. It speaks to the inherent desire within each of us to realise our fullest potential, to live our lives with intention and purpose. This pursuit is not governed by the external markers of success that society often champions. Rather, it is measured by the yardstick of personal growth, the depth of one's character, and the breadth of one's impact on the world.

The path to self-mastery is as diverse as the individuals who walk it. There is no one-size-fits-all approach, no prescriptive method that guarantees success. Each journey is unique, shaped by the individual's experiences, aspirations, and innate qualities. What remains constant, however, is the underlying framework that supports this endeavour: a commitment to continual learning, the cultivation of self-awareness, and the application of one's learnings in a way that harmonises with one's values and goals.

Engaging in this process of self-mastery requires a shift in perspective. It calls for viewing challenges not as obstacles, but as opportunities for growth. It necessitates a move away from a fixed mindset, where abilities are seen as static and predetermined, to a growth mindset, where the focus is on potential and the belief that effort and persistence can lead to improvement. This shift is not merely cognitive; it is deeply transformative, touching every aspect of one's life and reshaping one's understanding of what is possible.

Another cornerstone of self-mastery is emotional intelligence. The ability to recognise, understand, and manage one's own emotions, as well as to empathise with the emotions of others, is crucial. Emotional intelligence enhances our relationships, improves our decision-making, and allows us to navigate social complexities with finesse. Developing this aspect of mastery involves a delicate balance of introspection and engagement, requiring us to look inward to understand our emotional landscapes, while also looking outward to appreciate the perspectives and feelings of those around us.

The journey towards mastery is also a physical one. The state of our bodies can profoundly affect our mental and emotional well-being. Thus, attending to our physical health through proper nutrition, exercise, and rest is not ancillary to the process of self-mastery; it is integral. A healthy body supports a healthy mind, providing the energy and vitality needed to pursue our goals with vigour.

Mindfulness and meditation offer powerful tools for cultivating awareness and presence. These practices anchor us in the present moment, enabling us to observe our thoughts and emotions without judgement. This heightened state of awareness is liberating, allowing us to choose our responses to the world around us rather than being driven by unconscious patterns or impulses.

The pursuit of mastery also involves the development of practical skills and competencies. Whether it's mastering a craft, excelling in a profession, or acquiring new knowledge, the process of learning and skill acquisition is a testament to our capacity for growth and adaptation. It is a reminder that we are always in a state of becoming, always on the verge of discovering new depths to our abilities and new dimensions to our selves.

Yet, mastery is not solely an inward journey. It finds its fullest expression in the way we engage with the world. It involves building relationships that are rooted in authenticity and mutual respect, contributing to our communities in ways that are meaningful and impactful, and leading by example, inspiring others to embark on their own journeys of self-discovery and growth.

In embarking on this path, we must be prepared to

encounter resistance, both from within and without. The journey towards self-mastery challenges us to step out of our comfort zones, to confront our fears and insecurities, and to question long-held beliefs and assumptions. It requires resilience, the ability to bounce back from setbacks and failures, and the perseverance to continue moving forward, even when progress seems slow or uncertain.

This process of continuous self-improvement and personal growth is not a linear one. It is marked by cycles of expansion and contraction, progress and regression. There will be moments of profound insight and moments of doubt, times when the path ahead seems clear and times when it feels obscured by clouds of uncertainty. Yet, it is precisely this dynamic nature of the journey that makes it so enriching and transformative. Each step forward, each obstacle overcome, adds to our understanding of ourselves and enhances our ability to navigate the complexities of life.

One of the most significant challenges on the path to self-mastery is the tendency to be overly critical of oneself. In our pursuit of excellence, it is all too easy to fall into the trap of perfectionism, setting unrealistically high standards and berating ourselves when we fail to meet them. Cultivating self-compassion is crucial in this regard. It involves treating ourselves with the same kindness, understanding, and forgiveness that we would offer to a good friend. It means recognising that failure and imperfection are part of the human condition, and that growth often comes from our ability to learn from our mistakes, not from our ability to avoid them.

Another vital aspect of self-mastery is the ability to adapt to change. Life is inherently unpredictable, and the only constant is change itself. Developing flexibility and agility, the capacity to adjust our plans and strategies in response to changing circumstances, is essential. It requires us to be proactive, to anticipate potential challenges and opportunities, and to remain open to new ideas and perspectives.

Ultimately, the journey towards self-mastery is a deeply rewarding one. It offers the opportunity to live a life that is aligned with our deepest values and aspirations, to realise our potential, and to make a positive impact on the world around us. It is a path that leads to a deeper sense of satisfaction and fulfillment, to relationships that are richer and more meaningful, and to a sense of peace and contentment that comes from knowing we are living our lives to the fullest.

As we embark on this journey, it is important to remember that self-mastery is not a destination, but a process. It is not something to be achieved and then forgotten, but a way of being, a continuous practice that unfolds over the course of a lifetime. Each day offers a new opportunity to practice mastery, to learn something new about ourselves and the world, and to take another step towards becoming the individuals we aspire to be.

In this spirit, I invite you to approach this book not as a manual to be followed rigidly, but as a companion on your journey. Let it inspire you, challenge you, and guide you as you navigate the path towards self-mastery. Remember, the journey is as important as the destination, and every step taken in the spirit of growth and self-discovery is a step towards a more fulfilled and meaningful life.

May this journey bring you closer to the essence of who you truly are, and may you find joy, wisdom, and fulfillment in the process of becoming a master of yourself.

Embarking upon a journey of self-mastery begins with a crucial step: self-assessment. This process, fundamental to understanding one's current position in the vast landscape of personal development, involves a deep and often challenging exploration of one's strengths and weaknesses. It is through this exploration that we can chart a course towards growth, improvement, and ultimately, mastery over ourselves.

Self-assessment is not merely an exercise in self-evaluation but a nuanced process that requires honesty, introspection, and a willingness to confront both our greatest assets and our most challenging deficiencies. It is akin to holding a mirror up to one's soul, not for the sake of vanity but for the purpose of genuine reflection and understanding. This reflection is the first step towards crafting a blueprint for personal development, one that is tailored to the unique contours of one's individual character and circumstances.

The process of identifying one's strengths is often met with a mixture of pride and discomfort. On one hand, acknowledging our strengths allows us to recognise and celebrate the aspects of ourselves that contribute positively to our lives and the lives of others. It reinforces our sense of self-worth and provides a foundation upon which we can build. On the other hand, it requires us to confront the possibility that, in leaning too heavily on these strengths, we may have neglected other areas of potential growth.

Strengths come in myriad forms, often

categorised into talents (innate abilities), skills (abilities developed through practice), and knowledge (information acquired through learning). Identifying them requires a multifaceted approach, one that combines self-reflection with feedback from others. Reflective practices such as journaling or meditation can provide valuable insights into the situations in which we feel most competent and confident. Similarly, seeking feedback from friends, family, and colleagues can offer an external perspective on our abilities, highlighting strengths we may have overlooked or underestimated.

Conversely, the identification of weaknesses is a process fraught with vulnerability. It demands not only the courage to acknowledge our limitations but also the resilience to view them not as insurmountable barriers but as opportunities for growth. Weaknesses, much like strengths, can manifest in various aspects of our personality, skills, and knowledge base. They are not, however, immutable flaws but rather areas where our development has yet to reach its full potential.

The key to a productive assessment of weaknesses lies in the ability to approach them with a mindset of constructive criticism rather than self-reproach. This involves framing weaknesses in the context of potential improvement rather than inherent deficiency. For example, rather than viewing a lack of confidence in public speaking as a personal failing, it can be seen as an area for development, with specific steps that can be taken to improve.

The techniques for evaluating one's abilities and areas for improvement are as diverse as the individuals employing them. One effective method is the SWOT analysis, traditionally used in business contexts but equally applicable to personal development. This framework encourages individuals to identify their Strengths and Weaknesses (internal factors) and consider the Opportunities and Threats (external factors) that may impact their journey towards self-mastery. By mapping out these elements, one can develop a more holistic view of their personal landscape, identifying areas for improvement and strategies to leverage their strengths.

Another valuable technique is the use of psychometric assessments and personality tests. Tools such as the Myers-Briggs Type Indicator (MBTI) or the StrengthsFinder assessment offer insights into one's personality traits and innate strengths. While these tools should not be taken as definitive representations of one's character, they can provide a useful starting point for self-reflection and discussion.

Perhaps the most critical aspect of self-assessment, however, is the development of an action plan. Identifying strengths and weaknesses is only the first step; the true work lies in leveraging this knowledge towards personal growth. This involves setting specific, measurable, achievable, relevant, and time-bound (SMART) goals for improvement, identifying resources for learning and development, and establishing a system for tracking progress and reflecting on learning.

The journey of self-assessment is an ongoing one, a cyclical process of reflection, action, and evaluation. It requires a commitment to continuous learning and an openness to change, qualities that are essential for anyone seeking to master themselves. Through this process, we can develop a deeper understanding of our capabilities, foster a growth mindset, and take meaningful steps towards realising our full potential.

In conclusion, the process of self-assessment is a cornerstone of self-mastery. It provides the foundation upon which we can build a journey of personal development, one that is informed by a clear understanding of our strengths and weaknesses. By approaching this process with honesty, openness, and a commitment to growth, we can unlock the door to a deeper understanding of ourselves and embark on a path towards becoming the masters of our own destinies.

In the realm of self-improvement and personal development, the art of setting personal goals stands as a cornerstone practice, pivotal for anyone venturing towards the mastery of themselves. This chapter delves into the intricate process of crafting achievable aspirations that not only resonate with one's innermost desires but also serve as guiding stars on the journey to self-fulfilment and actualisation.

The initiation of setting personal goals demands a profound understanding of what truly motivates and moves us. It requires an introspective dive into the depths of our aspirations, unearthing the genuine ambitions that lie buried beneath the layers of societal expectations and external pressures. This exploration is not a trivial endeavour; it is an intimate dialogue with oneself, a conversation that necessitates honesty, vulnerability, and courage.

Emerging from this introspection should be a clearer vision of what we seek to achieve in various facets of our lives—be it in our careers, personal relationships, health and well-being, or personal growth. This vision acts as a beacon, illuminating the path forward and helping to align our daily actions with our deeper purpose. However, the mere identification of these aspirations is but the first step in a more elaborate process.

The transformation of these aspirations into tangible goals requires them to be distilled into specific, measurable, achievable, relevant, and time-bound (SMART) objectives. This methodology ensures that our goals are not mere figments of wishful thinking but attainable targets that challenge us to stretch beyond our current confines while remaining within the realm of possibility.

Specificity in goal setting eliminates ambiguity, providing a clear direction for our efforts. Measurability allows for the tracking of progress, offering tangible evidence of our advancements and areas needing improvement. Achievability ensures that while our goals push us to grow, they remain within the bounds of our capabilities, requiring perhaps a stretch but not a leap into the impossible. Relevance ties our goals to our core values and long-term objectives, ensuring that each step taken is in harmony with our overall life path. Lastly, time-bound goals imbue the journey with a sense of urgency and a deadline, compelling us to take action rather than succumb to procrastination.

Yet, the setting of goals, even when meticulously crafted, is not a guarantee of their fruition. The bridge between goal setting and goal achievement is built with the bricks of planning, discipline, and perseverance. It requires the construction of a detailed action plan that outlines the steps necessary to move from where we are to where we wish to be. This plan acts as a roadmap, guiding our daily actions and decisions towards the achievement of our goals.

Discipline, then, becomes the vehicle by which we traverse this path. It is the quality that enables us to adhere to our plan, to persist in our efforts even when faced with distractions, temptations, or setbacks. Discipline demands a commitment to our goals that supersedes the fleeting desires of the moment, a steadfastness that is unwavering in the face of challenges.

Perseverance, on the other hand, is what sustains us through the inevitable ups and downs of this journey. It is the resilience to bounce back from failures, to learn from our mistakes, and to continue pressing forward even when progress seems slow or non-existent. Perseverance recognises that the path to any worthwhile goal is seldom straight or smooth but is convinced of the value of the destination, regardless of the difficulties encountered along the way.

Integral to the process of goal setting and achievement is also the practice of reflection and adjustment. Regularly revisiting our goals allows us to assess our progress, celebrate our successes, and identify areas where adjustments may be necessary. It acknowledges that as we evolve, so too may our goals and aspirations, necessitating a flexibility in our approach and a willingness to recalibrate our path as needed.

Moreover, the journey towards our goals is not meant to be a solitary endeavour. The support and encouragement of others can be invaluable, providing motivation, accountability, and advice. Whether through formal mentorship, the camaraderie of like-minded individuals, or the support of friends and family, the involvement of others enriches the journey, adding layers of connection and shared experience.

In embracing the art of setting personal goals, we embark on a quest not just towards the achievement of specific objectives, but towards a deeper understanding of ourselves and our potential. It is a process that challenges us to define what we truly desire, to confront the barriers that stand in our way, and to cultivate the discipline and perseverance needed to overcome them. Through this process, we not only move closer to the realization of our goals but also to the mastery of ourselves.

As we journey forth, let us do so with clarity, conviction, and an open heart, ready to embrace the challenges and opportunities that lie ahead. Let us set our goals not as distant dreams, but as beacons of possibility, guiding us towards a future crafted by our own hands, a testament to the power of intention, effort, and self-mastery. In this endeavour, may we find not just success in the achievement of our goals but also growth in the journey towards them, discovering along the way facets of our character that were previously hidden and strengths that were untapped.

This journey of goal setting and achieving is inherently dynamic, reflecting the ever-evolving nature of human aspiration and capability. As we progress, our understanding of what is possible expands, and with it, our goals may shift and evolve. This is not a sign of failure or indecision, but rather an indication of growth and an increased awareness of our potential and desires. The ability to adapt our goals as we evolve is a crucial skill, ensuring that what we pursue remains aligned with our true selves and our changing circumstances.

Embracing the challenges that come

with pursuing our goals is also essential. These challenges are not mere obstacles but opportunities for learning and self-improvement. Each challenge faced and overcome is a step forward in our journey of self-mastery, a testament to our resilience and determination. They teach us about our limitations and how to push beyond them, about the value of persistence, and the importance of adaptability.

Moreover, the process of striving towards our goals can bring to light the significance of the journey itself. While the achievement of our goals is undoubtedly rewarding, it is the lessons learned, the skills acquired, and the person we become along the way that are of lasting value. This journey shapes us, moulding us into individuals capable of setting and achieving even greater aspirations in the future.

It is also through this process that we learn the importance of balance and well-being. The pursuit of our goals should not come at the expense of our health, relationships, or peace of mind. Instead, it should be integrated into a balanced life, where care for oneself and others is not overlooked in the single-minded pursuit of objectives. Achieving this balance is itself a goal, requiring mindfulness and intentionality in how we allocate our time and energy.

In conclusion, the art of setting and achieving personal goals is a fundamental aspect of the journey towards self-mastery. It challenges us to clarify our desires, confront our limitations, and engage in the disciplined pursuit of our aspirations. Through this process, we not only advance towards our chosen objectives but also embark on a profound journey of personal growth and discovery. As we navigate this path, let us remain open to the lessons it offers, embracing both the challenges and the joys it brings. In doing so, we not only move closer to achieving our goals but also to realising our fullest potential, crafting lives of purpose, meaning, and fulfilment.

In the vast and intricate tapestry of self-development, the cultivation of a mindset conducive to growth and resilience emerges as a pivotal endeavour, one that underpins the entire journey towards self-mastery. This chapter seeks to explore the nuances of fostering such a mindset, illuminating the pathways through which individuals can transform their perspective, embrace the ethos of continuous improvement, and navigate the inevitable ebbs and flows of life with grace and fortitude.

At the heart of a growth-oriented mindset lies the fundamental belief in the potential for change and development. Unlike a fixed mindset, which views talent and intelligence as static and unchangeable, a growth mindset thrives on the premise that abilities can be developed through dedication and hard work. This perspective not only opens the door to endless possibilities for learning and advancement but also instils a sense of agency and empowerment in the face of challenges.

Embracing a growth mindset, however, is not merely a matter of intellectual assent; it requires a profound and often challenging shift in how we perceive ourselves and our capabilities. It entails moving beyond the comfort zones of our existing beliefs and confronting the deeply ingrained narratives that may limit our perception of what is achievable. This process is inherently uncomfortable, demanding not only introspection but also the courage to question and, when necessary, dismantle those narratives.

One of the first steps in cultivating a growth mindset is to recognise and challenge the self-imposed limitations that stem from a fixed mindset. These limitations often manifest as a fear of failure, a reluctance to take on challenges, or a tendency to attribute success to innate talent rather than effort and perseverance. By acknowledging these tendencies, individuals can begin to reframe their approach to learning and achievement, viewing challenges not as threats but as opportunities for growth and development.

Central to the adoption of a growth mindset is the redefinition of failure. In a culture that often stigmatises mistakes and setbacks, adopting a perspective that sees failure as an integral part of the learning process is both revolutionary and liberating. It involves shifting the focus from outcomes to effort, recognising that setbacks are not reflections of inherent incapacity but rather stepping stones on the path to mastery. This reorientation fosters resilience, enabling individuals to persist in the face of difficulties and to extract valuable lessons from their experiences.

Moreover, the cultivation of a growth mindset is inextricably linked to the practice of self-compassion. The journey towards self-improvement is fraught with challenges and setbacks, and it is all too easy to succumb to self-criticism and discouragement. Practising self-compassion involves treating oneself with the same kindness, understanding, and patience that one would offer to a friend, recognising that imperfection is part of the human condition and that growth is a gradual and often nonlinear process.

Another cornerstone of developing a growth mindset is the commitment to lifelong learning. In a world that is constantly changing, the pursuit of knowledge and skill acquisition is not only a means of personal enhancement but also a strategy for remaining adaptable and relevant. Lifelong learning encompasses not only formal education but also informal learning opportunities, such as reading, engaging in new experiences, and seeking feedback and mentorship. It is characterised by curiosity, openness to new ideas, and a willingness to venture beyond the familiar.

The process of fostering a growth mindset also necessitates a reevaluation of how success is defined and measured. In a society that often equates success with external achievements and accolades, shifting the focus to personal progress and effort represents a significant paradigm shift. It involves setting personal benchmarks for success based on individual goals and values, celebrating small victories along the way, and recognising the intrinsic satisfaction derived from the pursuit of excellence.

Furthermore, cultivating a growth mindset involves embracing the power of yet. The word "yet" signifies the gap between current abilities and potential, offering a reminder that learning and growth are ongoing processes. This simple linguistic shift can transform perceptions of ability, turning statements of limitation into affirmations of possibility and underscoring the belief in the capacity for development and change.

The journey towards adopting a growth mindset is, by its very nature, iterative and evolving. It requires persistence, patience, and a willingness to embrace discomfort as a catalyst for transformation. Along the way, there may be moments of doubt and regression, but these, too, are part of the process, offering opportunities for reflection and recalibration.

In essence, the cultivation of a growth mindset is not merely a strategy for achieving specific goals but a fundamental orientation towards life. It is a commitment to viewing oneself and one's capabilities not as fixed entities but as works in progress, continually shaped by experiences, efforts, and the pursuit of learning. This perspective not only enhances personal resilience and adaptability but also enriches the journey of self-mastery, imbuing it with a sense of purpose, dynamism, and infinite possibility.

As we navigate the complexities of personal development, let us embrace the ethos of a growth mindset, recognising that within each of us lies the potential for change, improvement, and mastery. Let us approach challenges with curiosity and courage

, view setbacks as opportunities for learning, and celebrate our progress, however incremental, with joy and gratitude. In doing so, we not only advance towards our individual goals but also contribute to a culture that values growth, resilience, and the boundless potential of the human spirit.

In the exploration of self-mastery, one encounters the profound realm of time management, a discipline pivotal for harnessing one's most valuable resource: time. Mastery over this elusive and finite asset stands as a cornerstone in the edifice of personal development, enabling individuals to lead lives of purpose, productivity, and peace. This chapter delves into the intricacies of effective time management, offering insights into how one might navigate the ebb and flow of daily commitments with grace and efficacy, thereby unlocking the full spectrum of their potential.

At its essence, time management transcends the mere allocation of hours; it is the art of aligning one's actions with their deepest values and aspirations. It requires a discerning appraisal of how one's moments are spent, a commitment to prioritising what truly matters, and the cultivation of habits that facilitate focus and efficiency. In the journey towards self-mastery, the adept management of time is not an optional skill but a fundamental practice, one that enables individuals to carve out space for their pursuits amidst the cacophony of daily demands.

The first step in mastering time involves a rigorous assessment of one's current relationship with it. This necessitates an honest examination of how one allocates their hours, distinguishing between activities that are purposeful and those that are merely habitual or reactionary. Such an evaluation often reveals that much of our time is consumed by tasks that do not contribute to our overarching goals or well-being, be it through procrastination, distraction, or the acquiescence to others' demands on our time. Recognising these patterns is the first step towards reclaiming control over how our time is spent.

Following this assessment, the establishment of clear, purposeful goals emerges as a critical endeavour. These goals serve as beacons, guiding our allocation of time and ensuring that our actions are aligned with our values and aspirations. The act of setting goals imbues our daily tasks with meaning, transforming them from mere items on a to-do list into steps on the path to fulfilment. Moreover, it provides a framework for prioritisation, enabling us to discern between what is urgent and what is important, and to allocate our time accordingly.

The implementation of effective time

management strategies is, however, fraught with challenges, chief among them the lure of distraction. In an age where information is ubiquitous and attention is fragmented, the ability to focus has become a scarce commodity. Overcoming distraction requires not only the cultivation of discipline but also the creation of an environment conducive to concentration. This may involve the delineation of specific times and spaces for work, the use of tools that limit access to distractions, and the practice of mindfulness, allowing one to remain present and engaged with the task at hand.

Moreover, effective time management necessitates the embrace of flexibility. While the establishment of routines and schedules can enhance productivity, an overly rigid approach to time can lead to frustration and burnout. Life is inherently unpredictable, and the ability to adapt to changing circumstances while maintaining focus on one's goals is a hallmark of true mastery over time. This flexibility allows us to respond to the unexpected with grace, adjusting our plans without losing sight of our priorities.

Another key aspect of time management is the practice of delegation and the willingness to say no. In our efforts to meet expectations and fulfil obligations, we often take on more than we can reasonably manage. Learning to delegate tasks that can be handled by others, and to decline requests that do not align with our goals or values, is essential for preserving our time for what truly matters. This not only enhances our own productivity but also empowers those around us, fostering a sense of trust and collaboration.

The art of time management also involves the recognition and honouring of our natural rhythms. Each individual has times of day when they are most alert and creative, as well as times when their energy wanes. By aligning our tasks with these rhythms, scheduling demanding work during our peak periods and less intensive tasks during our lulls, we can maximise our efficiency and the quality of our output.

In the pursuit of effective time management, the role of rest and rejuvenation cannot be overstated. Far from being a mere cessation of activity, rest is an active and vital component of productivity, allowing for the replenishment of our mental and physical reserves. It is in the spaces between our activities that insights emerge, creativity flourishes, and we reconnect with our deeper selves. Thus, the management of time is not merely about doing more but about achieving a balance that fosters both productivity and well-being.

In conclusion, the mastery of time management is a multifaceted endeavour, requiring self-awareness, discipline, and a commitment to living in accordance with one's values. It is about making conscious choices, each day, about how we spend our most precious resource, ensuring that our actions reflect our deepest aspirations. Through the thoughtful allocation of our time, we not only enhance our productivity and achieve our goals but also carve out space for the things that bring us joy, fulfilment, and a sense of purpose. In mastering time, we step closer to mastering ourselves, navigating the journey

 of life with intention, grace, and a profound appreciation for each moment granted to us.

Crafting the foundation upon which all aspects of personal development rest requires a deep engagement with the concept of discipline. Often misconstrued as a punitive measure or a restrictive force, discipline, in its essence, is the bedrock of freedom and self-mastery. It is the structured approach to harnessing one's energies, directing them towards the realisation of goals and the cultivation of a life of purpose and fulfilment. This chapter unfolds the layers of discipline, shedding light on its transformative power and offering guidance on how to integrate this pivotal practice into the fabric of one's daily life.

At its core, discipline is the practice of making consistent choices that align with one's values and long-term objectives, even in the face of immediate temptations or distractions.

It is the art of self-regulation, a deliberate effort to mould one's behaviour and habits in service of greater aspirations. Discipline is not about the suppression of desire but the alignment of desire with that which is genuinely enriching and meaningful. It requires a nuanced understanding of one's motivations, strengths, and weaknesses, as well as the development of strategies to navigate the complexities of human will and desire.

The journey towards cultivating discipline begins with the establishment of clear, compelling goals. These goals act as lighthouses, guiding individuals through the fog of daily distractions and providing a sense of direction and purpose. However, the setting of goals is merely the first step; the crux of discipline lies in the commitment to taking regular, consistent actions towards these goals. It is the daily choices, the small acts of self-control, and the incremental progress that weave the fabric of a disciplined life.

One of the most significant challenges in the practice of discipline is the management of procrastination and distraction. In an era where distractions are incessantly vying for our attention, the capacity to focus on what truly matters becomes increasingly rare and valuable. Overcoming these challenges necessitates an understanding of the triggers that lead to procrastination and the development of strategies to mitigate them. This may involve the structuring of one's environment to minimise distractions, the use of tools and techniques to enhance focus, and the cultivation of mindfulness, enabling a deeper engagement with the present moment and the task at hand.

Moreover, discipline is closely linked to the concept of habit formation. Habits, the automatic behaviours that constitute a significant portion of our daily lives, have the power to propel us towards our goals or to lead us astray. The conscious cultivation of positive habits, therefore, is a cornerstone of discipline. This process involves the identification of keystone habits, those core routines that have a disproportionate impact on our lives, and the implementation of strategies to reinforce these habits until they become ingrained in our daily practice.

The role of motivation in the cultivation of discipline cannot be overstated. While discipline can propel us forward even in the absence of motivation, finding sustainable sources of motivation can enhance our resilience and perseverance. This involves connecting with the deeper why behind our goals, understanding the intrinsic rewards of our endeavours, and celebrating the milestones along the journey. It is the interplay between discipline and motivation that fuels our progress, enabling us to overcome obstacles and to persist in the face of adversity.

Another critical aspect of discipline is the management of energy. Recognising that our mental, emotional, and physical energies are finite and fluctuating resources is essential. Effective discipline involves not only the regulation of our actions but also the stewardship of our energy, ensuring that we allocate our resources in a manner that is sustainable and aligned with our priorities. This may involve the adoption of practices that replenish our energy, such as rest, exercise, and mindfulness, as well as the establishment of boundaries to protect our time and well-being.

Furthermore, the journey towards a disciplined life is not a solitary endeavour. The support of a community, the guidance of mentors, and the accountability provided by peers can significantly enhance our capacity for discipline. These relationships offer encouragement, inspiration, and a sense of shared purpose, reinforcing our commitment to our goals and to the practice of discipline itself.

In essence, discipline is a form of self-love, a commitment to honouring one's potential and to the cultivation of a life that is reflective of one's deepest values and aspirations. It is not a destination but a continuous process, a series of choices made each day, in each moment. Through the practice of discipline, we not only achieve our goals but also discover a greater sense of self-mastery, autonomy, and fulfilment.

As we navigate the complexities of life, let us embrace discipline not as a burden but as a liberating force, a means through which we can realise our full potential and craft lives of purpose and meaning. In the disciplined pursuit of our aspirations, we find not only the achievement of our goals but also the transformation of our character, the deepening of our resolve, and the unfolding of our truest selves.

In the pursuit of self-mastery, the cultivation of positive habits stands as a monumental pillar, essential for steering one's life towards greater fulfilment, productivity, and well-being. Habits, the often-overlooked automatic actions performed daily, shape the very fabric of our existence, quietly running in the background, dictating the rhythm and direction of our lives. This chapter delves into the profound impact of habits on personal development, unravelling the process of habit formation and offering insights on how to consciously craft habits that align with one's aspirations and values.

At the outset, it's crucial to acknowledge the dual nature of habits: while some propel us towards our goals, acting as catalysts for growth and progress, others may tether us to past limitations, hindering our journey towards self-improvement. The key, therefore, lies in the deliberate cultivation of positive habits and the mindful attenuation of those that no longer serve our purpose. This endeavour, while seemingly daunting, is imbued with the potential to transform one's life from the mundane to the extraordinary.

The genesis of habit formation lies in understanding the psychological framework that underpins it. Habits are formed through a loop process that begins with a cue, followed by a routine, and culminating in a reward. The cue triggers the behaviour, the routine is the behaviour itself, and the reward is the benefit derived from the behaviour. Recognising this cycle provides a blueprint for dismantling undesired habits and fostering beneficial ones. By identifying the cues that lead to negative routines and substituting them with positive actions that lead to equally or more rewarding outcomes, one can gradually reshape their habitual landscape.

Embarking on the journey of habit formation demands an initial investment of effort and willpower. However, as positive habits become ingrained, they start to require less conscious energy, seamlessly integrating into the fabric of daily life. The establishment of keystone habits, those which have a ripple effect, catalysing a series of positive changes across various aspects of life, is particularly transformative. For instance, the habit of regular exercise not only enhances physical health but also promotes mental clarity, emotional stability, and a sense of discipline that permeates other areas of life.

The environment plays a pivotal role in the formation and sustenance of habits. A conducive environment, tailored to support specific habits, significantly lowers the barrier to engagement. For example, a workspace organised and designated solely for work-related tasks can enhance productivity and focus. Similarly, removing temptations and distractions from one's immediate environment can facilitate the adherence to habits that require greater self-control, such as studying or dietary restrictions.

Accountability and social support further bolster habit formation. Sharing one's goals and desired habits with a supportive community or accountability partner can provide the external motivation needed to maintain consistency, especially during moments of waning internal motivation. The encouragement and feedback from others not only foster a sense of shared endeavour but also amplify the commitment to the habit formation process.

Reflection and adjustment are integral to the habit cultivation journey. Regularly reviewing one's habits, assessing their alignment with personal goals, and making necessary adjustments ensures that habits remain relevant and supportive of one's evolving aspirations. This reflective practice encourages a proactive stance towards personal development, fostering a dynamic and responsive approach to habit formation.

Moreover, patience and self-compassion are essential companions on the path to establishing new habits. Given the deeply ingrained nature of some behaviours, immediate transformation is unrealistic. Acknowledging this and approaching habit formation with patience, accepting setbacks as part of the learning process, and treating oneself with kindness and understanding can make the journey more sustainable and rewarding.

The ultimate aim of habit formation is not just the automation of positive actions but the cultivation of a lifestyle that resonates with one's deepest values and aspirations. It's about creating a life where the default actions contribute to a sense of progress, well-being, and fulfilment. Through the deliberate shaping of our habits, we wield the power to sculpt our lives into masterpieces of our own design, reflecting our highest potentials and deepest convictions.

In essence, the art of habit formation is a testament to the remarkable capacity for self-directed change inherent in each individual. It underscores the profound truth that, through the accumulation of small, consistent actions, we have the power to transform our lives radically. As we navigate the complexities of personal development, let us embrace the transformative power of habits with intentionality and vigour. Let the conscious cultivation of positive habits be the vehicle through which we journey towards the pinnacle of self-mastery, crafting lives of purpose, joy, and unparalleled fulfilment.

In the intricate dance of personal development, emotional intelligence emerges as a profound and pivotal skill, a beacon guiding individuals through the complex web of human emotions and interactions. This chapter seeks to delve deep into the essence of emotional intelligence, unravelling its components and exploring the transformative impact it has on our lives, relationships, and the pursuit of self-mastery.

Emotional intelligence, at its core, is the capacity to recognise, understand, manage, and utilise emotions effectively in ourselves and others. It is a multifaceted skill, encompassing self-awareness, self-regulation, motivation, empathy, and social skills. These components, woven together, form a tapestry that enriches our understanding of the human experience, enhancing our ability to navigate the seas of personal and professional life with grace, resilience, and understanding.

The journey towards cultivating emotional intelligence begins with self-awareness, the cornerstone of this profound skill. Self-awareness involves an intimate understanding of our emotions, their triggers, and their effects on our thoughts and behaviours. It demands a reflective and introspective approach, a willingness to delve into the depths of our inner world and confront the truths that lie within. This self-exploration, though often challenging, illuminates the patterns of our emotional responses, granting us the insight needed to foster growth and change.

Building upon the foundation of self-awareness, self-regulation comes into play as the capacity to manage and direct our emotions in a healthy and constructive manner. It is the skill that allows us to pause between feeling and action, choosing responses that align with our values and goals rather than being swept away by the tempest of immediate emotions. Self-regulation involves techniques such as mindfulness, cognitive restructuring, and the practice of adaptive coping strategies, enabling us to maintain equilibrium in the face of life's inevitable challenges and stresses.

Motivation, another key facet of emotional intelligence, is the drive that propels us towards our goals, fuelled by a deep understanding of our emotional landscape. It involves harnessing our emotions in service of our aspirations, transforming them into a source of energy and persistence. Motivated individuals are characterised by their resilience, their capacity to remain optimistic and focused in the pursuit of long-term objectives, even when faced with setbacks and obstacles.

Empathy, the ability to perceive and understand the emotions of others, stands as a pillar of emotional intelligence, enriching our connections and interactions. It extends beyond mere sympathy, involving an active engagement with the emotional experiences of others, fostering a sense of understanding, compassion, and connection. Empathy enhances our ability to communicate effectively, navigate conflicts, and build deep, meaningful relationships, both personally and professionally.

Lastly, social skills, the outward expression of emotional intelligence, encompass our ability to interact, influence, and build rapport with others. It involves adeptly navigating social situations, resolving conflicts, inspiring and leading, and fostering positive relationships. Social skills are built upon the foundation of self-awareness, self-regulation, motivation, and empathy, culminating in a sophisticated understanding of social dynamics and the ability to navigate them with tact and grace.

The cultivation of emotional intelligence is not a destination but a journey, a continuous process of learning, growth, and adaptation. It requires a commitment to self-exploration, the willingness to confront and understand our emotions, and the dedication to applying this understanding in our interactions with others. The benefits of this endeavour are profound, touching every aspect of our lives. Emotionally intelligent individuals enjoy deeper relationships, greater personal and professional success, and a heightened sense of well-being and fulfilment.

Moreover, emotional intelligence plays a critical role in the realm of leadership and influence. Leaders equipped with emotional intelligence inspire trust, empathy, and motivation in their teams, fostering environments where creativity, collaboration, and productivity flourish. They navigate the complexities of human dynamics with understanding and strategic insight, driving positive change and innovation.

In essence, emotional intelligence is the golden thread that weaves together the fabric of our lives, enriching our experiences, enhancing our relationships, and empowering us to navigate the world with confidence and compassion. It is a testament to the profound impact of understanding and managing our emotions, a skill that transforms not only our lives but also the lives of those around us.

As we journey towards self-mastery, let us embrace the cultivation of emotional intelligence with open hearts and minds, recognising its transformative power and its pivotal role in our personal and professional development. Let us commit to the continuous exploration of our emotional landscape, fostering a deep, nuanced understanding of ourselves and others. In doing so, we unlock the full potential of our humanity, stepping into a world of greater connection, understanding, and fulfilment.

In the voyage towards achieving a harmonious and balanced life, the significance of integrating the physical self with the mental and emotional spheres cannot be overstated. This chapter aims to explore the profound interconnection between physical health and well-being and its undeniable influence on our journey towards self-mastery and personal fulfilment. It delves into the necessity of nurturing our bodies, not merely as vessels through which we navigate the world but as integral components of our very essence, deeply entwined with our mental and emotional states.

The foundation of this holistic approach lies in the recognition that the mind and body are not separate entities but parts of a singular, interconnected system. The state of our physical health exerts a profound influence on our mental clarity, emotional resilience, and overall capacity for personal growth. Conversely, our mental and emotional well-being can significantly impact our physical health, creating a cyclical relationship that underscores the importance of addressing both aspects in our quest for self-improvement.

Central to nurturing the physical self is the practice of regular physical activity. Exercise, beyond its widely acknowledged health benefits, serves as a powerful catalyst for mental and emotional well-being. Engaging in physical activity releases endorphins, the body's natural mood elevators, which can alleviate symptoms of stress and depression, enhance cognitive function, and foster a sense of overall well-being. Moreover, the discipline and commitment required to maintain a consistent exercise regimen can reinforce our willpower and self-control, key attributes in the pursuit of self-mastery.

Equally important is the role of nutrition in maintaining optimal physical and mental health. The food we consume directly affects our brain's structure and function, and consequently, our moods and energy levels. A diet rich in nutrients supports cognitive processes, emotional balance, and physical vitality, empowering us to engage more fully in our personal development efforts. Conversely, poor dietary habits can lead to a decline in both physical and mental health, hampering our ability to achieve our goals and realise our potential.

Rest and recovery, too, are pivotal in the integration of the physical self. In our fast-paced, often relentless pursuit of success, the value of rest is frequently overlooked. Yet, adequate sleep and periods of rest are crucial for cognitive function, emotional resilience, and physical health. Sleep serves as a period of regeneration, during which the body repairs itself, and the mind consolidates memories and processes emotions. Insufficient rest not only impairs our physical health but also our cognitive abilities, emotional stability, and productivity, highlighting its indispensable role in our overall well-being.

Furthermore, the practice of mindfulness and meditation offers a bridge between the physical and mental realms. These practices encourage a heightened state of awareness and presence, allowing us to tune into our bodily sensations and emotional states. Through mindfulness, we can cultivate a deeper understanding of the connection between our physical experiences and our mental and emotional reactions, fostering a sense of inner harmony and balance.

The pursuit of physical well-being, however, extends beyond individual practices to encompass our broader lifestyle choices and environments. The spaces in which we live and work, the quality of the air we breathe, and our engagement in recreational activities all contribute to our physical health and, by extension, our mental and emotional well-being. Creating environments that nurture our physical selves can amplify our efforts towards personal growth, enhancing our capacity for self-mastery.

In embracing the integration of the physical self, it is essential to adopt a compassionate and flexible approach. Our bodies, like our minds, are subject to fluctuations and changes, requiring us to adjust our practices and expectations accordingly. Cultivating an attitude of self-compassion and patience towards our physical limitations and needs can enhance our resilience and encourage a more sustainable approach to personal development.

In conclusion, the journey towards self-mastery and personal fulfilment is intrinsically linked to the state of our physical health and well-being. By nurturing our bodies through exercise, nutrition, rest, and mindfulness, we not only enhance our physical vitality but also our mental clarity, emotional resilience, and overall capacity for growth. The integration of the physical self is not merely a component of personal development but a fundamental pillar upon which the edifice of self-improvement is built. As we continue on our path towards achieving a balanced and harmonious life, let us honour and nurture our physical selves, recognising their vital role in our quest for self-mastery and the realisation of our fullest potential.

Venturing into the realms of mindfulness and meditation reveals a transformative pathway towards achieving a deeper understanding of oneself, enhancing focus, and cultivating a serene mind amidst the tumultuous landscapes of modern life. This exploration into the quietude of being offers not only a refuge from the relentless pace of daily activities but also serves as a foundational practice in the journey towards self-mastery. Embracing mindfulness and meditation facilitates a profound connection with the present moment, allowing for an enriched appreciation of life's experiences and fostering a resilient, peaceful state of mind.

Mindfulness, in its essence, is the practice of being fully present and engaged with the here and now, without judgment. It involves a conscious awareness of our thoughts, feelings, bodily sensations, and the surrounding environment, observed from a place of detachment and curiosity. This practice encourages a shift in perspective, enabling individuals to witness their internal landscapes without being ensnared by them. It cultivates a space where thoughts and emotions can be acknowledged without criticism, allowing for a compassionate understanding of oneself and a recognition of the transient nature of our experiences.

The incorporation of mindfulness into daily life begins with simple, yet profound, practices. It might start with the mindful observation of one's breath, noticing the inhalation and exhalation, the rise and fall of the chest, and the sensation of air moving through the nostrils. This basic practice can serve as an anchor, bringing the mind back to the present whenever it wanders into the territories of the past or the future. Gradually, mindfulness can extend beyond breath awareness to include mindful eating, walking, and listening, transforming routine activities into opportunities for presence and connection.

Meditation, often intertwined with mindfulness, offers a structured approach to cultivating a quiet and focused mind. It encompasses a variety of practices, including concentration meditation, where focus is maintained on a single point of reference, and insight meditation, which encourages an open awareness of all aspects of the present moment. Meditation provides a space for the mind to rest, free from the constant stimulation of external inputs, leading to increased mental clarity, emotional stability, and a deeper sense of inner peace.

The benefits of a regular mindfulness and meditation practice are manifold, extending far beyond the immediate experience of relaxation. Over time, practitioners often report enhanced emotional intelligence, increased empathy, and a greater capacity for compassion towards themselves and others. These practices can also mitigate the effects of stress, anxiety, and depression, contributing to overall well-being and mental health. Furthermore, mindfulness and meditation have been shown to improve concentration and cognitive function, enabling individuals to navigate the complexities of life with greater ease and efficiency.

Incorporating mindfulness and meditation into one's life does not necessitate lengthy sessions or retreats into solitude. The beauty of these practices lies in their accessibility and adaptability to various lifestyles and needs. Even brief periods of meditation or mindful awareness integrated into the daily routine can yield significant benefits. The key is consistency and the intention to cultivate a deeper awareness and presence in each moment.

The path towards integrating mindfulness and meditation into daily life begins with setting realistic expectations and a gentle, non-judgmental approach towards oneself. It is a journey marked by patience, as the fruits of these practices often unfold gradually over time. Encounters with restlessness, resistance, and distraction are common and serve as valuable opportunities to deepen one's practice, offering insights into the workings of the mind and the art of returning to the present.

As one delves deeper into the practice of mindfulness and meditation, a transformation begins to take shape, not only in moments of quietude but in the very fabric of daily life. This transformation is characterised by a heightened sense of connection to oneself and the world, a deepened capacity for joy and gratitude, and an enhanced resilience in the face of life's inevitable challenges. The practices of mindfulness and meditation thus emerge not merely as tools for personal development but as essential components of a life lived with depth, purpose, and clarity.

In essence, the journey into mindfulness and meditation is an invitation to explore the landscapes of the mind, to cultivate a sanctuary of peace within, and to engage with the world from a place of grounded presence and awareness. It is a pathway towards self-mastery that beckons with the promise of a more conscious, connected, and compassionate existence. As we venture forth on this journey, let us embrace the practice of mindfulness and meditation with openness and curiosity, allowing it to illuminate our path towards a life of greater awareness, serenity, and fulfilment.

Navigating through life's inevitable challenges and setbacks requires more than just a positive attitude; it necessitates a comprehensive strategy for resilience and adaptation. This chapter unfolds the essence of overcoming obstacles, transforming them from seemingly insurmountable barriers into opportunities for growth and development. The journey towards self-mastery is punctuated with moments of difficulty and adversity, yet it is precisely within these moments that the potential for significant personal growth lies. Embracing challenges as catalysts for change can lead to profound insights and a deeper understanding of one's strengths and capabilities.

At the heart of overcoming obstacles is the cultivation of resilience, the ability to bounce back from setbacks with increased strength and wisdom. Resilience is not an innate trait bestowed upon a select few but a skill that can be developed and strengthened over time. It involves a dynamic interplay between maintaining a positive outlook, fostering emotional regulation, and adopting a flexible approach to problem-solving. Building resilience requires a conscious effort to focus on what can be controlled, letting go of the frustration associated with factors beyond one's influence.

A pivotal step in transforming obstacles into opportunities is the practice of reframing, a cognitive technique that involves changing the way one perceives a challenge. Reframing is not about denying the difficulty of a situation but about viewing it from a perspective that highlights potential growth and learning. By shifting focus from the obstacle itself to the skills and knowledge that can be gained from addressing it, individuals can find motivation and purpose even in the face of adversity. This shift in perspective is crucial for maintaining momentum towards one's goals, preventing the stagnation that often accompanies a fixed or negative mindset.

Emotional regulation plays a critical role in navigating through challenges. The initial response to a setback often involves a surge of emotions such as frustration, disappointment, or fear. Recognising and accepting these emotions without becoming overwhelmed by them is essential for clear thinking and effective decision-making. Techniques such as deep breathing, mindfulness, and positive self-talk can aid in managing emotional responses, allowing for a more rational and constructive approach to problem-solving.

Flexibility and adaptability are further key components in overcoming obstacles. Life's unpredictability demands a willingness to adjust one's course of action in response to new information or changing circumstances. This flexibility involves letting go of rigid expectations and remaining open to alternative paths towards one's goals. It is through this adaptability that individuals can navigate around obstacles, finding creative solutions and discovering new opportunities that may not have been apparent initially.

The support of a strong social network is invaluable in the face of challenges. Sharing one's experiences with trusted friends, family, or mentors can provide not only emotional support but also different perspectives and advice. The encouragement and understanding of others can be a powerful source of strength, reminding individuals that they are not alone in their struggles. Furthermore, witnessing the resilience of others can serve as a source of inspiration and motivation.

Learning from failure is an integral part of overcoming obstacles. Each setback provides a unique opportunity for introspection and analysis, allowing individuals to identify what went wrong and how similar challenges can be approached differently in the future. This process of reflection and learning fosters a growth mindset, wherein failure is seen not as a reflection of one's worth but as a stepping stone towards success.

Finally, maintaining a sense of purpose and keeping sight of one's long-term goals is essential during times of difficulty. Obstacles can often lead to feelings of disillusionment or a loss of direction. Reconnecting with the reasons behind one's pursuits can reignite motivation and provide the clarity needed to persevere. It is the alignment with one's values and the pursuit of meaningful objectives that lend the strength and determination to overcome any obstacle.

In conclusion, the ability to navigate through and overcome obstacles is a testament to one's resilience, adaptability, and strength of character. By embracing challenges as opportunities for growth, employing strategies for emotional regulation and problem-solving, and drawing on the support of a strong social network, individuals can transform setbacks into stepping stones towards self-mastery. The journey may be fraught with difficulties, but it is within these moments of adversity that the potential for profound personal growth and transformation lies. Let us approach each obstacle with courage, determination, and an unwavering belief in our ability to emerge stronger and more resilient on the other side.

In the landscape of personal development, the art of communication stands as a pivotal skill, bridging the gap between individuals, fostering understanding, and enhancing relationships. This chapter delves into the intricate dance of exchanging ideas, emotions, and information, highlighting the transformative power of effective communication on our journey towards self-mastery.

At its essence, communication is the lifeblood of human connection, a complex interplay of verbal and non-verbal cues, active listening, and empathetic response. It involves not only the transmission of messages but also the reception and interpretation of those messages, a reciprocal process requiring attentiveness, openness, and sensitivity to the nuances of human interaction.

The foundation of effective communication lies in the cultivation of active listening, a skill that extends beyond the mere auditory reception of words to encompass a deep engagement with the speaker's message. Active listening involves fully concentrating on what is being said, understanding the underlying emotions and intentions, and responding in a way that validates the speaker's perspective. This practice not only enhances the quality of interactions but also builds trust and rapport, creating a safe space for open and honest dialogue.

Empathy plays a crucial role in effective communication, serving as a bridge to understanding and connection. It involves the ability to see the world through another's eyes, to feel what they feel, and to communicate that understanding back to them. Empathy enriches our interactions, enabling us to respond to others with compassion, sensitivity, and a genuine interest in their well-being. It is through empathetic communication that we can navigate conflicts with grace, foster deeper relationships, and create a sense of community and belonging.

Clarity and conciseness are further key elements of effective communication. In a world inundated with information, the ability to convey messages clearly and succinctly is invaluable. This involves choosing words carefully, structuring thoughts logically, and avoiding ambiguity. Clear communication reduces the potential for misunderstanding, ensuring that our ideas and intentions are accurately received and understood.

Non-verbal communication, encompassing body language, facial expressions, and tone of voice, adds a rich layer of meaning to our interactions. These cues can reinforce or contradict the verbal message, offering insights into emotions and attitudes that words alone may not convey. Being mindful of our non-verbal signals, and attuning to those of others, can enhance the depth and authenticity of our communications, revealing the unspoken elements of our interactions.

The skill of assertiveness is integral to effective communication, enabling individuals to express their thoughts, needs, and boundaries clearly and respectfully. Assertiveness is not about dominance or aggression but about the confidence to voice one's opinions and the respect for the right of others to do the same. It fosters a balanced dialogue where all parties feel heard and valued, facilitating constructive exchanges and mutual understanding.

Adaptability and cultural sensitivity are essential for navigating the diverse landscape of human interaction. Recognising that communication styles can vary widely across different cultures and contexts, and adjusting our approach accordingly, can prevent misunderstandings and foster harmonious relationships. It involves an awareness of cultural norms and values, a willingness to learn and adapt, and a respect for diversity in all its forms.

In the pursuit of self-mastery, the development of communication skills is not merely a tool for effective interaction but a pathway to deeper self-understanding and personal growth. It challenges us to listen more deeply, to empathise more fully, and to express ourselves with greater clarity and confidence. Through the practice of effective communication, we can navigate the complexities of human relationships with finesse, build meaningful connections, and contribute positively to the world around us.

In conclusion, the art of communication is a cornerstone of personal development, a skill that enriches our lives and the lives of those with whom we interact. By fostering active listening, empathy, clarity, and assertiveness, and by being mindful of non-verbal cues and cultural sensitivities, we can enhance our ability to connect with others, resolve conflicts, and build strong, supportive relationships. As we journey towards self-mastery, let us embrace the power of communication, recognising it as a vital instrument in our toolkit for personal and professional growth.

Embarking on the journey of financial mastery is a critical aspect of self-improvement and personal development. It transcends the mere accumulation of wealth, focusing instead on cultivating a mindset that values financial responsibility, strategic planning, and the pursuit of financial freedom. This chapter aims to unravel the complexities of achieving financial mastery, offering insights into how one can navigate the path towards financial independence and security, thereby enhancing overall quality of life and enabling the pursuit of one's true passions and goals.

Financial mastery begins with the development of financial literacy, a fundamental understanding of financial principles, practices, and the dynamics of the economy. It involves educating oneself about budgeting, saving, investing, and the wise management of debt. This foundational knowledge is crucial for making informed decisions that align with one's financial goals and aspirations, thereby laying the groundwork for long-term financial stability.

At the heart of financial mastery lies the art of budgeting, a practice that enables individuals to gain control over their finances by tracking income, managing expenses, and setting aside savings. Effective budgeting is not about restriction but about making conscious choices, prioritising spending in ways that reflect one's values and long-term objectives. It requires discipline and foresight, qualities that are essential for navigating the financial landscape with confidence and precision.

Saving and investing emerge as pivotal components of financial mastery, mechanisms through which one can build wealth over time. Saving provides a safety net, a reserve for unforeseen expenses and emergencies, while investing offers the potential for wealth accumulation through the strategic allocation of assets. Understanding the principles of investment, including the balance between risk and return, asset diversification, and the power of compound interest, is vital for crafting a robust investment strategy that can weather the uncertainties of the market.

Debt management is another critical aspect of financial mastery. In a world where debt has become a ubiquitous part of financial life, learning to manage and reduce debt is essential for financial health. This involves understanding the cost of debt, prioritising the repayment of high-interest debts, and utilising strategies that minimise the burden of debt over time. Effective debt management not only alleviates financial stress but also enhances one's capacity to invest in future opportunities.

Beyond these practical aspects, financial mastery also requires a shift in mindset, a move away from short-term gratification towards long-term financial well-being. It involves cultivating a sense of delayed gratification, recognising that the sacrifices made today can lead to substantial rewards in the future. This mindset shift is crucial for overcoming the temptations of consumer culture and for focusing on achieving financial goals that bring lasting satisfaction and security.

Financial mastery also encompasses the ability to adapt to changing financial circumstances, maintaining flexibility in one's financial planning to accommodate life's unpredictabilities. This adaptability is key to navigating financial challenges and opportunities with agility, ensuring that one's financial strategy remains aligned with evolving goals and circumstances.

Moreover, achieving financial mastery involves understanding the broader impact of one's financial decisions, including their social and environmental implications. Ethical investing, socially responsible spending, and the support of businesses and practices that align with one's values are expressions of financial mastery that extend beyond personal gain, contributing to the well-being of the community and the planet.

In the pursuit of financial mastery, it is essential to approach the journey with patience and perseverance. Financial independence and security are not achieved overnight but are the result of consistent, mindful efforts over time. It requires a commitment to continuous learning, self-reflection, and the willingness to make adjustments as needed.

In conclusion, financial mastery is a multifaceted endeavour that plays a crucial role in personal development and self-mastery. It involves cultivating financial literacy, practising disciplined budgeting, saving and investing wisely, managing debt effectively, and adopting a long-term perspective towards financial well-being. By embracing the principles of financial mastery, individuals can achieve financial independence, reduce stress, and create a foundation for pursuing their true passions and goals. As we navigate the path towards financial mastery, let us do so with diligence, foresight, and a commitment to making financial decisions that enrich our lives and the world around us.

In the grand tapestry of personal development, the cultivation of creative thinking emerges as a vibrant thread, enriching the fabric of our lives with innovation, problem-solving capabilities, and an enhanced appreciation for the complexity of the world around us. This chapter delves into the essence of creative thinking, exploring how one can foster this invaluable skill to unlock new perspectives, overcome challenges, and bring a fresh dynamism to their personal and professional endeavours.

Creative thinking is not confined to the realms of artistry or invention alone but is a universal skill that can be nurtured across all aspects of life. It involves breaking free from conventional thought patterns to explore ideas and solutions that are original, unconventional, and reflective of one's unique perspective. At its core, creative thinking champions the idea that multiple solutions can exist for any given problem and that these solutions can be reached through a process of exploration, experimentation, and an open-minded approach to the unknown.

The journey towards enhancing creative thinking begins with cultivating an environment that encourages curiosity and open-ended inquiry. This involves embracing a mindset that values questions as much as answers, recognising that the pursuit of understanding is as important as the destination. Such an environment is not just physical but also psychological, one where individuals feel safe to express their thoughts and ideas without fear of judgement or failure.

Diversifying one's experiences is another fundamental strategy for fostering creative thinking. Exposure to different cultures, disciplines, and ways of life can significantly expand one's cognitive horizons, introducing new patterns of thought and perspectives that can inspire innovative ideas. This diversification can take many forms, from travelling and learning new languages to engaging with art, music, and literature from a wide array of genres and traditions.

The practice of brainstorming and ideation plays a crucial role in the development of creative thinking. This process encourages the generation of ideas without immediate critique or evaluation, allowing for a free flow of thoughts that can later be refined and assessed for feasibility. Techniques such as mind mapping, free writing, and lateral thinking exercises can stimulate the mind, revealing connections and possibilities that were previously obscured.

Critical to the nurturing of creative thinking is the acceptance of ambiguity and the willingness to tolerate uncertainty. Creative processes often involve navigating through periods of confusion and doubt, where the path forward is not clear. Embracing this uncertainty as a natural and necessary component of creativity allows for a more resilient and adaptable approach to problem-solving, where the journey through the unknown becomes a source of insight and innovation.

Collaboration and the exchange of ideas with others offer rich soil for the growth of creative thinking. Interaction with individuals from diverse backgrounds and with varying viewpoints can spark new ideas, challenge existing assumptions, and lead to the co-creation of solutions that are richer and more nuanced than those generated in isolation. The collaborative process underscores the principle that creativity thrives in spaces where dialogue, feedback, and the merging of perspectives are encouraged and valued.

In addition to these strategies, the cultivation of creative thinking requires the dedication of time and space for reflection and solitude. Moments of quiet introspection can be profoundly fertile grounds for creativity, providing the mind with the opportunity to wander, make novel connections, and incubate ideas. It is in these moments of stillness that insights often emerge, revealing new paths and possibilities that were previously hidden from view.

Furthermore, the nurturing of creative thinking involves a conscious effort to overcome the fear of failure. The creative process is inherently experimental, entailing a degree of risk and the possibility of mistakes. Viewing these mistakes not as setbacks but as integral steps in the journey towards innovation can significantly reduce the anxiety associated with creative endeavours, fostering a more playful, adventurous approach to problem-solving.

In conclusion, the enhancement of creative thinking is an enriching endeavour that transcends the boundaries of artistic expression, permeating every facet of personal and professional life. It involves the cultivation of an inquisitive mindset, the diversification of experiences, the practice of brainstorming and collaboration, and the acceptance of ambiguity and failure as part of the creative process. By embracing these principles, individuals can unlock their creative potential, bringing a sense of innovation, flexibility, and depth to their pursuits. As we navigate the complexities of the modern world, let us champion creative thinking as a vital skill, one that empowers us to envision and realise a future that is not only possible but also imbued with possibility, originality, and transformative potential.

The essence of building a personal brand transcends the mere construction of a public persona; it delves into the articulation of one's authentic self, values, and visions, crafting a narrative that resonates deeply with both oneself and the broader audience. This chapter explores the journey of personal branding, a journey that intertwines self-discovery with strategic communication, aiming to establish a distinctive and genuine identity in the vast tapestry of the modern world.

Personal branding is not about donning a facade or projecting what we presume others wish to see; rather, it is the strategic articulation of our authentic selves, our unique blend of skills, experiences, and passions. It's about finding our voice and using it to communicate our values and vision to the world. In doing so, we not only carve out our niche but also attract the opportunities and connections that align with our genuine self.

At the heart of personal branding lies the process of self-discovery, a reflective journey that demands honesty and introspection. It requires us to ask ourselves profound questions: Who am I? What do I stand for? What are my passions and strengths? How do I wish to impact the world? The answers to these questions form the foundation of our brand, guiding the narrative we wish to share with the world.

Once clarity on one's identity and values is achieved, the next step involves the articulation of this personal brand. This articulation is not limited to verbal communication but extends to all forms of expression, from the way we dress and present ourselves to our online presence and the content we create. Every interaction and piece of content becomes a brush stroke in the larger painting of our personal brand, each contributing to a cohesive and authentic image.

In the digital age, the internet and social media platforms offer unparalleled opportunities to project and amplify our personal brand. However, navigating this digital landscape requires strategic thinking and a consistent effort to ensure that our online presence aligns with the authentic identity and values we wish to convey. It's about curating content that reflects our expertise, passions, and the unique value we offer, engaging with our audience in a way that fosters genuine connections and community.

Networking, both online and offline, plays a crucial role in the development and dissemination of our personal brand. It's about forging connections not just for the sake of expanding our professional network but for building meaningful relationships with individuals who share our values and vision. Effective networking involves active listening, empathy, and the mutual exchange of value, principles that are at the core of meaningful personal and professional relationships.

The journey of personal branding also encompasses the continuous process of learning and growth. As we evolve, so too does our brand. It's a dynamic entity that reflects our journey, achievements, and the ever-expanding horizon of our aspirations. Staying open to new experiences, continuously honing our skills, and adapting our brand to reflect our growth are essential for maintaining relevance and resonance with our audience.

Moreover, the practice of authenticity in personal branding cannot be overstated. In a world saturated with curated images and narratives, authenticity stands out as a beacon of integrity and genuineness. It's about being true to ourselves and our vision, even when it means standing apart from the crowd. Authenticity fosters trust and loyalty, creating a deep and lasting impact on those we reach.

In conclusion, building a personal brand is a profound journey of self-discovery and strategic expression, a journey that allows us to articulate our unique identity and values in a way that resonates with others. It involves clarity of purpose, consistent communication, strategic use of digital platforms, meaningful networking, continuous growth, and unwavering authenticity. As we navigate this journey, we not only carve out our niche but also create a legacy that reflects our true selves, attracting opportunities and connections that enrich both our personal and professional lives. Let us embrace the journey of personal branding with courage, creativity, and authenticity, crafting a narrative that is not only distinctive but deeply true to who we are and aspire to be.

Navigating the intricate web of personal and professional relationships stands as a pivotal chapter in the journey towards self-mastery. The art of cultivating and sustaining meaningful connections requires more than mere social skills; it demands an understanding of the nuanced dynamics of human interactions, empathy, and a commitment to genuine engagement. This exploration delves into the essence of building and nurturing relationships that not only enrich our lives but also foster personal growth and a sense of community.

At the core of meaningful relationships is the concept of authenticity. Authentic interactions are the bedrock upon which trust and intimacy are built, allowing for a connection that transcends superficial exchanges.

Being authentic means showing up as our true selves, without the facades that we often hide behind in social situations. This vulnerability, while daunting, invites others to engage with us on a deeper level, fostering relationships grounded in honesty and mutual respect.

Empathy, the ability to understand and share the feelings of another, is another cornerstone of meaningful relationships. It enables us to see the world through the eyes of others, to connect with their experiences on an emotional level, and to respond with compassion and understanding. Empathy bridges the gap between diverse perspectives and experiences, creating a space for mutual support and connection. It is through empathetic engagement that we can truly appreciate the complexity of those around us, paving the way for relationships that are rich in understanding and solidarity.

Active listening is a critical skill in the cultivation of relationships. It involves fully concentrating on what is being said, understanding the message, responding thoughtfully, and remembering the information shared. Active listening demonstrates respect and interest in the speaker, validating their experiences and feelings. It is a powerful tool for building rapport and trust, essential components of any strong relationship.

The maintenance of relationships requires effort and intentionality. It involves consistent communication, the sharing of experiences, and the willingness to invest time and energy into the relationship. This commitment signals the value we place on our connections with others, reinforcing the bonds that tie us together. Regular check-ins, celebrating achievements, offering support during challenges, and sharing moments of joy and sorrow are all practices that strengthen relationships over time.

Conflict resolution skills are indispensable in the realm of relationships. Disagreements and misunderstandings are inevitable in any human interaction, but the manner in which they are addressed can either harm or enhance the relationship. Approaching conflicts with a mindset of finding a mutually beneficial resolution, employing effective communication strategies, and maintaining respect for the other party are key to navigating disputes constructively. Viewing conflicts as opportunities for growth and deeper understanding can transform them from divisive experiences into catalysts for strengthening the relationship.

The art of giving and receiving feedback is another aspect of building meaningful relationships. Constructive feedback, delivered with care and respect, can be a gift that promotes personal and professional growth. Similarly, being open to receiving feedback, even when it is challenging, demonstrates humility and a commitment to self-improvement. The exchange of feedback, when done within the context of a supportive relationship, can deepen trust and facilitate mutual development.

Finally, the expansion of one's social circle through networking offers opportunities to build new relationships and strengthen existing ones. Networking, however, should not be viewed merely as a means to an end but as an opportunity to connect with like-minded individuals, share knowledge and experiences, and contribute to a community. Genuine networking is characterised by a desire to build relationships based on mutual interests and respect, rather than solely for personal gain.

In conclusion, the journey towards cultivating and sustaining meaningful relationships is a multifaceted endeavour that enriches our personal and professional lives. It requires authenticity, empathy, active listening, commitment, effective conflict resolution, and the ability to give and receive feedback. By embracing these principles, we can build a network of connections that supports our journey towards self-mastery, offering companionship, inspiration, and a sense of belonging. As we navigate the complexities of human relationships, let us do so with an open heart and a commitment to genuine engagement, fostering connections that not only endure but also inspire and elevate.

The pursuit of contributing beyond oneself, to give back to the community and make a positive impact in the world, is a profound aspect of personal development and self-mastery. This chapter explores the significance of service and contribution, not as an afterthought to personal success, but as an integral part of a fulfilled and meaningful life. Engaging in acts of service and contribution not only enriches the lives of others but also enhances our own personal growth, happiness, and sense of purpose.

At the heart of contribution is the recognition of our interconnectedness and the understanding that our actions have the power to affect the lives of others. This awareness prompts a shift from a self-centric perspective to a broader, more inclusive view of our role in the world. It challenges us to look beyond our immediate concerns and consider how we can utilise our skills, resources, and time to make a positive difference in the lives of others.

Engaging in service and contribution begins with cultivating a mindset of generosity and empathy. It involves developing a genuine concern for the welfare of others and a willingness to act on that concern without expectation of reward or recognition. This mindset of generosity is not confined to financial giving but encompasses a wide range of actions, including volunteering time, sharing knowledge, and offering emotional support to those in need.

The benefits of engaging in acts of service and contribution are manifold. On a personal level, it fosters a sense of satisfaction and fulfilment that comes from knowing we have made a positive impact in the world. It can also provide a sense of connection and community, as we work alongside others towards a common goal. Moreover, service and contribution can offer new perspectives and insights, challenging us to grow and expand our understanding of the world and our place within it.

Identifying opportunities for service and contribution requires mindfulness and intentionality. It involves reflecting on our passions, skills, and the needs of our community to find areas where we can make a meaningful contribution. This reflection can lead to a wide range of activities, from volunteering at local charities and mentoring others, to engaging in environmental conservation efforts and advocating for social justice. The key is to find activities that resonate with our values and allow us to utilise our strengths in service of something greater than ourselves.

Overcoming barriers to service and contribution is an essential step in this journey. Time constraints, self-doubt, and a lack of awareness of opportunities can all hinder our ability to contribute. Addressing these barriers involves setting clear priorities, seeking out opportunities for engagement, and recognising that even small actions can have a significant impact. It also requires cultivating a belief in our own ability to make a difference, challenging the notion that one person's efforts cannot change the world.

The act of giving back and contributing

to the community also plays a crucial role in building leadership skills and personal resilience. It provides opportunities for problem-solving, teamwork, and navigating challenges, all of which contribute to personal and professional growth. Furthermore, service and contribution can inspire others to take action, creating a ripple effect of positive change that extends far beyond the initial act.

In conclusion, service and contribution are not merely adjuncts to personal development but are foundational elements of a life well-lived. They enrich our lives, enhance our connections with others, and provide a profound sense of purpose and fulfilment. By embracing the mindset of generosity and actively seeking opportunities to make a difference, we can contribute to a more compassionate, just, and sustainable world. As we continue on our journey of self-mastery, let us remember that the greatest measure of our success is not the accolades we receive, but the impact we have on the lives of others and the world we leave behind.

Embarking on the path towards adaptability and change is an essential chapter in the narrative of self-mastery and personal development. In a world characterised by constant flux, the ability to adapt, evolve, and embrace change not only as an inevitable but as a beneficial aspect of life, stands as a testament to personal resilience and flexibility. This exploration delves into the nuances of adaptability, shedding light on strategies for navigating change with grace, and transforming the challenges it presents into opportunities for growth and self-discovery.

Adaptability is the capacity to adjust one's thoughts, behaviours, and actions in response to new information, changing circumstances, or unexpected challenges. It involves a willingness to let go of old patterns that no longer serve us and to embrace new experiences with openness and curiosity. At its core, adaptability is about maintaining a balance between being firm in one's values and flexible in one's approach to life's ever-changing dynamics.

The foundation of adaptability lies in cultivating a growth mindset, a perspective that views challenges as opportunities to learn and evolve. This mindset encourages individuals to step out of their comfort zones, to experiment, and to see failure not as a setback but as a valuable part of the learning process. By fostering a growth mindset, we equip ourselves with the psychological resilience necessary to navigate the uncertainties of life with confidence and optimism.

Embracing change requires an acute

awareness of the impermanence of life's conditions. Recognising that change is the only constant allows us to detach from fixed expectations and to approach life with a sense of fluidity. This awareness can liberate us from the fear of the unknown, enabling us to view change not as a threat but as an invitation to grow and to explore new possibilities.

Building emotional resilience is crucial for thriving in times of change. It involves developing the inner resources needed to manage stress, to recover from adversity, and to maintain a sense of equilibrium amidst life's ups and downs. Emotional resilience can be nurtured through practices such as mindfulness, which fosters a non-reactive awareness of our thoughts and emotions, allowing us to respond to change with intention rather than being swept away by it.

Effective communication plays a pivotal role in adaptability, particularly in the context of relationships and teamwork. The ability to articulate one's needs, to listen to and consider the perspectives of others, and to negotiate solutions that accommodate changing circumstances is vital for navigating the social aspects of change. Clear, empathetic communication fosters collaboration and understanding, making the process of adaptation smoother and more inclusive.

Strategic planning and goal setting, while maintaining flexibility, are also key components of adaptability. Setting clear goals provides direction and purpose, guiding our actions even as we remain open to adjusting our plans in response to new information or opportunities. This balance between having a vision and being willing to modify it as needed is a hallmark of adaptive individuals.

Moreover, cultivating a network of support can provide the encouragement and assistance needed to manage change effectively. Surrounding ourselves with a diverse group of individuals who offer different perspectives and skills can enhance our ability to adapt, providing resources, advice, and encouragement when facing new challenges.

In conclusion, adaptability and the embrace of change are not merely survival strategies in an uncertain world but are essential qualities for personal growth and self-mastery. By cultivating a growth mindset, building emotional resilience, communicating effectively, and maintaining a flexible approach to goal setting, we can navigate the currents of change with agility and grace. As we continue on our journey of personal development, let us view change not as a barrier but as a pathway to discovering new horizons, expanding our capabilities, and evolving into our fullest selves.

Leadership and influence, when wielded with intention and integrity, transcend mere authority and control, evolving into powerful instruments for positive change, inspiration, and the collective achievement of shared visions. This exploration delves into the nuanced realms of leadership and influence within the context of self-mastery, elucidating how these attributes can be cultivated to not only guide others towards success but also to foster environments of collaboration, growth, and mutual respect.

Leadership, at its essence, is the ability to motivate, guide, and inspire individuals towards achieving a common goal. It is not confined to positions of formal authority but is a quality that can be manifested in every interaction and endeavour. True leadership is characterised by a commitment to serving others, by prioritising the well-being and development of the team over personal accolades or gains.

The journey towards becoming an effective leader begins with self-awareness, an understanding of one's strengths, weaknesses, values, and the impact of one's behaviour on others. This introspection lays the groundwork for authentic leadership, a style that is rooted in genuine intention, transparency, and a deep alignment with one's personal values. Authentic leaders inspire trust and loyalty, fostering an atmosphere where individuals feel valued, heard, and motivated to contribute their best.

Influence, closely intertwined with leadership, is the capacity to shape the perspectives, attitudes, and actions of others. It extends beyond mere persuasion, encompassing the ability to connect with others on a deeper level, to understand their needs and aspirations, and to align these with the broader objectives. Influence is built on the foundations of credibility, trust, and respect, qualities that are earned through consistent actions, empathy, and a genuine commitment to the welfare of others.

Empowering others is a hallmark of effective leadership and influence. It involves recognising and nurturing the potential within individuals, providing them with the opportunities, resources, and support needed to grow and excel. Empowerment fosters a sense of ownership and responsibility, encouraging innovation and initiative, and contributing to a culture of excellence and accountability.

Effective communication is paramount in the exercise of leadership and influence. It encompasses not only the clear articulation of ideas and expectations but also active listening and the ability to engage in meaningful dialogue. Through effective communication, leaders can build consensus, navigate conflicts, and articulate a compelling vision that galvanises the team towards common objectives.

Adaptability and flexibility are critical attributes for leaders and influencers navigating the complexities of the modern world. The ability to adjust strategies, embrace new ideas, and remain resilient in the face of challenges is essential for guiding teams through uncertain times. Adaptive leaders are characterised by their openness to learning, their willingness to pivot when necessary, and their capacity to inspire confidence and maintain morale even under adverse conditions.

Finally, the practice of ethical leadership and influence is non-negotiable. It involves making decisions that are aligned with ethical principles and standards, demonstrating integrity, and setting an example for others to follow. Ethical leaders and influencers earn the trust and respect of their teams, laying the foundation for sustainable success and a legacy of positive impact.

In conclusion, leadership and influence, when cultivated within the framework of self-mastery, offer profound opportunities to effect positive change, inspire excellence, and contribute to the collective well-being. By embracing authenticity, empowering others, communicating effectively, adapting to change, and upholding ethical standards, individuals can ascend to leadership and influence roles that not only achieve goals but also elevate those around them. As we navigate our personal and professional journeys, let us aspire to be leaders and influencers who enrich the lives of others, fostering environments where collaboration, growth, and mutual respect flourish.

The conclusion of a journey towards self-mastery and personal development is not a destination but a continuous cycle of growth, reflection, and evolution. As we venture through the various chapters of self-improvement—embracing change, honing our communication skills, leading with integrity, and contributing to the world around us—we uncover the profound truth that the journey itself is where the true transformation occurs. This exploration does not culminate in a final chapter but rather in the understanding that each step taken, each challenge faced, and each insight gained is part of an ongoing process of becoming our best selves.

Self-mastery is an art that requires patience, perseverance, and a deep commitment to continuous learning. It is about embracing our imperfections, celebrating our progress, and always striving towards a greater understanding of ourselves and the world around us. The pursuit of personal development is driven by an inner desire to live a life of purpose, to make a meaningful impact, and to realise our fullest potential.

One of the key insights from this journey is the recognition that self-mastery is not a solitary endeavour. It is enriched and deepened by our interactions with others—our mentors, peers, and the community at large. The relationships we cultivate along the way not only support and inspire us but also challenge us to grow and expand our perspectives. Through collaboration, empathy, and mutual support, we discover that our capacity to learn and evolve is limitless.

Moreover, the pursuit of self-mastery teaches us the value of resilience and adaptability. Life's inevitable challenges and setbacks are not obstacles but opportunities to develop our inner strength, to practice grace under pressure, and to emerge more robust and wise. It is through facing adversity with courage and an open heart that we learn the true extent of our capabilities and discover the power of a positive, growth-oriented mindset.

The journey towards self-mastery also highlights the importance of living authentically and with intention. By aligning our actions with our values and aspirations, we create a life that is not only fulfilling but also a true reflection of who we are. Authenticity breeds trust, connection, and a sense of peace, allowing us to navigate the complexities of life with integrity and purpose.

As we continue on this path, it is essential to remember that self-mastery is an ever-evolving process. What we learn and achieve today lays the foundation for future growth, inspiring us to pursue new goals, to embrace new challenges, and to continue expanding our horizons. The journey of personal development is infinite, with each chapter building upon the last, guiding us towards greater understanding, compassion, and fulfilment.

In conclusion, the journey towards self-mastery and personal development is a profound and enriching experience that shapes every aspect of our lives. It challenges us to grow, to connect deeply with others, and to contribute positively to the world. As we navigate this journey, let us do so with curiosity, courage, and an unwavering commitment to becoming our best selves. The path of self-improvement is not linear but a spiral of continuous growth, where each turn reveals new vistas of possibility and potential. Let us embrace this journey with open hearts and minds, knowing that the pursuit of self-mastery is not just about reaching a destination but about savouring the journey itself, with all its twists, turns, and revelations.

As we draw the curtains on this exploration of self-mastery and personal development, we stand at a juncture that reflects both an ending and a beginning. The final chapter of this journey is not a signal to halt but a beacon inviting us to continue venturing deeper into the realms of self-discovery, growth, and transformation. It's a moment to pause, reflect, and appreciate the distance travelled, while also gazing forward into the horizon, where new challenges and opportunities await.

The path towards self-mastery is etched with the footprints of our trials, triumphs, and the invaluable lessons gleaned along the way. Each chapter we've navigated has equipped us with knowledge, skills, and insights to foster a life of purpose, fulfilment, and contribution. Yet, the essence of this journey lies in the recognition that self-mastery is an ever-evolving quest, a lifelong commitment to learning, evolving, and striving towards the embodiment of our highest potential.

As we move forward, let us carry with us the understanding that the journey of personal development is inherently personal and unique. There is no one-size-fits-all roadmap or definitive endpoint; rather, it's a mosaic of experiences, reflections, and actions that are deeply individual and continuously unfolding. Embracing this journey requires courage to face the unknown, resilience to weather the storms, and an open heart to learn from every experience, whether it be joyous or challenging.

The pursuit of self-mastery is underpinned by a series of choices—

choices to grow, to change, to persevere, and to live authentically. It's about choosing to rise each day with intention, to act in alignment with our values, and to embrace each moment as an opportunity for growth. This journey teaches us the power of our agency, reminding us that we are the architects of our destiny, capable of shaping our lives through the decisions we make and the actions we take.

As we forge ahead, it's essential to remember that self-mastery is not a solitary endeavour but a journey enriched by the connections we share with others. The relationships we cultivate, the communities we build, and the contributions we make to the world around us are integral to our growth and fulfilment. These connections remind us of our shared humanity, offering support, inspiration, and a sense of belonging that fuels our journey.

The final chapter of this book is but a comma in the ongoing narrative of our lives, a pause before the next chapter begins. It's an invitation to continue exploring, learning, and growing, to remain curious and open to the endless possibilities that life offers. The path of self-mastery is boundless, and with each step, we uncover new layers of ourselves, new challenges to overcome, and new horizons to explore.

In closing, let us embrace the journey of self-mastery with gratitude for the lessons learned, courage for the challenges ahead, and the unwavering belief in our ability to evolve and thrive. May we continue to seek out growth, to inspire and be inspired, and to live our lives with purpose, passion, and perseverance. The journey of self-mastery is a testament to the indomitable spirit of the human heart, a journey that enriches not only our lives but also the world around us.

As we turn the page, let us step forward with confidence, curiosity, and a deep commitment to the never-ending journey of becoming our best selves. The path ahead is ours to shape, and the journey of self-mastery, with all its twists and turns, is a journey worth embracing in its entirety.

I